A
Clinical Thinking

Barbara Bates, MD

Clinical Professor of Medicine
Medical College of Pennsylvania

Clinical Professor of Nursing
University of Pennsylvania School of Nursing
Philadelphia, Pennsylvania

J.B. Lippincott Company
Philadelphia

Sponsoring Editor: Donna L. Hilton, RN, BSN
Coordinating Editorial Assistant: Susan M. Keneally
Ancillary Coordinator: Doris S. Wray
Copyeditor: Mary Norris
Compositor: Richard G. Hartley
Printer/Binder: R.R. Donnelly & Sons Co., Crawfordsville

ISBN: 0-397-55249-1

6   5

Any procedure or practice described in this book should be
applied by the health care practitioner under appropriate
supervision in accordance with professional standards of care
used with regard to the unique circumstances that apply in
each practice situation. Care has been taken to confirm the
accuracy of information presented and to describe generally
accepted practices. However, the authors, editors, and pub-
lisher cannot accept any responsibility for errors or omissions
or for any consequences from application of the information
in this book and make no warranty, express or implied, with
respect to the contents of the book.

Every effort has been made to ensure drug selections and
dosages are in accordance with current recommendations and
practice. Because of ongoing research, changes in govern-
ment regulations, and the constant flow of information on
drug therapy, reactions, and interactions, the reader is cau-
tioned to check the package insert for each drug for the
indications, dosages, warnings, and precautions, particularly
if the drug is new or infrequently used.

Table of Contents

Gathering Data 3

   Taking a Comprehensive History . . . 3

      Elements of the History 4

      Attributes of a Symptom 6

   Performing a Physical Examination . . 7

Applying Clinical Thinking to the Data . 9

Developing a Problem List and a Plan 13

Creating the Patient's Record 14

Mrs. N.: A Case Study 15

   Mrs. N's Record 15

   Mr. N.'s Problem List and Plan . . . 25

Clinical Thinking is an invisible process but it will give visible shape to the data that you gather throughout your clinical interactions. From the moment you see a patient and listen to the chief complaints, you develop ideas about what may explain the complaints and how you can determine their probable nature and cause with increasing certainty. At the same time, you are learning about the patient as a person, the meaning of the illness to that person and perhaps to others, and its impact on their lives.

The thinking process continues as you gather a health history and perform a physical examination. Findings from each of these two sources can raise or lower the likelihood of certain problems or diagnoses. They may virtually exclude some of your initial ideas about what is wrong with the patient or open up new avenues for exploration.

As you start to learn the skills of taking or doing a physical examination, you may not be ready to do much clinical thinking. You are busy trying to remember what questions to ask or where to place your stethoscope. When practicing your skills with a laboratory partner, however, you may suspect an abnormality. If so, you will probably want to consult your instructor, but you can also start to develop your thinking skills. You will get further, more complicated opportunities to think clinically after taking comprehensive histories and doing more complete examinations.

With experience, you will gradually become able to alter the details of how you conduct your interview and examination as your findings unfold and their possible meanings are clarified. Your approach to a woman with hypertension will differ from your approach to a man with cough, fever and weight loss. Clinical thinking creates this difference.

Getting an overview of the sequence of clinical practice — from gathering data to making a plan with the patient — will help you to understand how each component of the process fits into the whole, as diagrammed below.

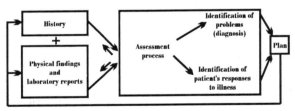

Note that this sequence is basically circular, and you may cycle through the process or through parts of the process as often as necessary.

Gathering Data

Essential to the thinking process are data to think about. In clinical practice, the data include symptoms, signs, and possibly laboratory reports. *Symptoms* are unusual physical or psychological feelings that the patient experiences and describes to you; you will record them in the patient's history. *Signs* are the physical or mental manifestations that you discover by physical examination; you will describe these in the patient's record as findings.

Taking a Comprehensive History

The way you talk with a patient while taking a history lays the foundation for good care. Listen carefully. Respond skillfully and empathically. Learn what is bothering the patient and what symptoms have been experienced. You may also learn what the patient thinks the trouble may be, how or why it happened, and what outcome is hoped for or feared. As you listen, begin to formulate a range of possible diagnoses. By asking additional questions, you can fill in the gaps in the patient's initial account and test some of your diagnostic hypotheses.

This process, if done well, develops your understanding of the patient and, in turn, helps the patient to feel both heard and understood — key elements in beginning to build as trusting relationship between you. What you learn while taking a history also helps to shape the history itself, and suggests the most relevant body parts or systems on which to focus your physical examination. At a later stage of care, it will affect your explanations to the patient and your shared plan for the future.

The items in a history vary with a patient's age, sex, and illness, with the clinician's specialty and available time, and with the goals of the visit. Although a limited approach, tailored to a particular problem, may be indicated, a comprehensive history is needed in other circumstances. Learn and understand all the items in such a history. If you master the full process, you will be able to select the items you need as your clinical and diagnostic skills improve and you begin to make informed choices.

Elements of the History

After listing introductory information about the patient, begin the main part of the history with the patient's **chief complaints** — the one or more symptoms or other concerns for which the patient is seeking care or advice. When possible, record these complaints in the patient's own words.

The **present illness** amplifies the chief complaints and, in its written form, gives a full, clear chronological account of how each of the symptoms developed and what events were related to them. It also includes how the patient thinks and feels about the problem or illness, how it has affected the patient's life and functions, and what concerns have led to seeking attention.

The chief complaints and the present illness are probably the most important parts of the history. Other components are significant:

- **Past history**:   prior illnesses, injuries, and medical interventions

- **Current health status**:   present state of health, and any environmental conditions, personal habits, and health-related measures that may impinge on it

- **Family history**:   a listing of outline that helps you to assess the patient's risks of developing certain diseases, may suggest what the patient is worried about, and may reveal a pattern of familial illness useful in the care of related persons

- **Psychosocial history**:   may suggest contributory factors in the patient's illness, may help you to evaluate the patient's sources of support, likely reactions to illness, coping mechanisms, strengths, and concerns, and may increase your understanding of the patient as a person

- **Review of systems**: questions about common symptoms in each major body system, which may help to identify problems that the patient has not mentioned

Note that there will be variations in the history in some areas when the patient is a child or an adolescent.

Attributes of a Symptom

The principal symptoms should be described in terms of the following attributes, which are building blocks of your diagnostic reasoning.

1. **Location**. Where is it? Does it radiate?

2. **Quality**. What is it like?

3. **Quantity or severity**. How bad is it?

4. **Timing**. When did (does) it start? How long does it last? How often does it come?

5. **Setting in which it occurs**, including environmental factors, personal activities, emotional reactions, or other circumstances that may have contributed to the problem

6. **Factors that make it better or worse**

7. **Associated manifestations**

Performing a Physical Examination

Examine the patient systematically, with special emphasis on areas suggested by the present illness and the chief complaints.

The categories of a physical examination include:

General survey
Vital signs
Skin
Head
Eyes
Ears
Nose and sinuses
Mouth and pharynx
Neck
Breasts and axillae
Thorax and lungs
Cardiovascular system
Abdomen
Genitalia
Anus and rectum
Peripheral vascular system
Musculoskeletal system
Nervous system
Mental status

As in the history, there will be variations in technique when you examine children.

Master the techniques involved in each area of the comprehensive examination before you begin to make informed omissions based on your developing skills in the clinical thinking. Be thoughtful about the patient's physical and psychological comfort with the various stages of the examination, and maintain friendly communication as you proceed. Be careful not to show dismay, or to be overly reassuring before all the data are in hand.

Applying Clinical Thinking to the Data

Given the data collected, whether partial or fairly complete, you can analyze any apparent problem by following these steps:

1. **Identify the abnormal findings**: symptoms, physical signs, and available laboratory test results.

2. **Cluster these findings into logical groups.**

3. **Localize the findings anatomically** as precisely as the data allow. This may be easy. For example, the symptoms of a scratchy throat and the sign of reddened pharynx clearly localize a problem in the pharynx. Other data may present difficulty. Chest pain, for example, can originate from many sources. Some symptoms and signs, such as fatigue and fever, have no localizing value but may be useful in the next step.

4. **Interpret the findings in terms of the probable process:**

   > *Pathological*, involving an abnormality in a body structure

Pathophysiological, involving an abnormality in a body function

Psychopathological, involving a disorder of mood or thinking

5. **Make one or more hypotheses about the nature of the patient's problem.**

- *Select the most specific and central findings around which to construct your hypothesis.* If a patient reports loss of appetite, nausea, vomiting, fatigue, and fever, for example, and if you find a tender, somewhat enlarged liver and mild jaundice, build your hypothesis around jaundice and hepatomegaly rather than fatigue or fever. Although the other symptoms are useful, they are much less specific.

- Using your inferences about structures and processes involved, *match your findings against all conditions you know can produce them.* For example, you can match the patient's red throat with a list of inflammatory conditions affecting the pharynx, or you can compare the symptoms and signs of the jaundiced patient with the various inflammatory, toxic, and neoplastic conditions that might produce this kind of clinical picture.

- *Eliminate the hypotheses that fail to explain the findings.* You might consider conjunctivitis as a cause of the patient's red eye, for example, but eliminate this possibility because it does not explain the dilated pupil or decreased visual acuity. Acute glaucoma would explain all these findings.

- *Weigh the probability of competing hypothesis* according to

    Their match with the findings

    The statistical probability of a given disease in a patient of this age, sex, race, habits, lifestyle, locality, and other variables

    The timing of the patient's illness

- *Consider carefully the possibility of potentially life-threatening and treatable conditions,* such as meningococcal meningitis, bacterial endocarditis, or subdural hematoma, even if they are less common and thus less likely.

6. **Test the hypothesis.** You may need further history, additional maneuvers on physical examination, or laboratory studies.

7. **Establish a working definition of the problem** at the highest level of explicitness and certainty that the data allow.

Developing a Problem List and a Plan

After you have made the best assessment of the patient's problems that you can from the data available, list the problems by name for the patient's record. Each problem may be considered active or inactive, and each should be dated and numbered.

The problem list will help you to organize a plan for the patient. For each active problem that needs attention, develop a plan that has three potential parts: diagnostic, therapeutic, and educational. Whenever possible, patients should participate in making this plan. Their goals, attitudes, economic means, and competing responsibilities will all affect the practicality, acceptability, and wisdom of the plan, and involving them from the beginning will improve everyone's chance of success.

Creating the Patient's Record

The patient's record documents your findings, your assessment of their nature and causes, your diagnostic conclusions, and your plan for the patient. The record should be accurate, clear, well, organized, and legible.

It should also emphasize important features and omit the irrelevant. Although making this distinction may be difficult, here are some guidelines:

- Record all the positive data that contribute to your assessment.

- Describe the negative data, e.g., the absence of a symptom or sign, when this affects your assessment.

- Data not recorded are data lost, but data buried in trivial details may be overlooked.

- Describe findings in positive terms, not in lists of negatives, e.g., "eardrum gray, intact," rather than "eardrum without redness or perforation."

- Avoid redundancies. Because resonance of the lungs can only be found on percussion, for example, omit "on percussion."

- And omit repetitive introductory phrases, e.g., "The patient reports no......."

Mrs. N.: A Case Study

Mrs. N's Record

Below is a clinician's record of a visit with Mrs. Audrey N., included here as an example of the process of a history and physical examination and how to record what is learned from them. A problem list and a plan will follow the record.

Mrs. Audrey N., 1463 Maple Blvd., Capital City

11/13/94

Mrs. N. is a 54-year-old, widowed, white saleswoman, born in the U.S.

Referral. None

Source. Self, seems reliable

Chief Complaint. Headaches

Present Illness. For about 3 mo increasingly troubled by headaches: bifrontal, usually aching, occasionally throbbing, mild to moderately severe. Has missed work only once because of headaches, when felt nauseated, and vomited several times — otherwise, nausea rare. Headaches now only average once a week, usually are present on waking and last all day. Relieved by lying down and using cold wet towel on head. Little relief from aspirin. No other related symptoms, no local weakness, no numbness or visual symptoms.

"Sick headaches" with nausea and vomiting began at age 15, recurred through her mid-20s, then diminished to one every 2 or 3 mo and almost disappeared.

Has recently had increased pressure at work from a new and demanding boss, and is also worried about her daughter (see psychosocial). Thinks headaches may be like those in past, but wants to be sure because mother died of stroke. Concerned that they make her irritable with her family

Past History

General health.   Good

Childhood Illnesses.   Only measles and chickenpox

Adult Illnesses.   Acute kidney infection, 1982, with fever and right flank pain treated with ampicillin. A generalized rash with itching developed several days later. Kidney x-rays said to be normal, and infection has not recurred.

Psychiatric Illness.   None

Injuries.   Stepped on glass at beach, 1991, laceration, sutured, healed

Operations.   Tonsillectomy, age 6; appendectomy, age 13

Current Health Status

Medications.   Aspirin for headaches, multivitamins. Has taken "water pill" for ankle swelling, but none in past several mo

*Allergies.   Ampicillin caused rash.

---

*   Underline or asterix important points.

Tobacco. About 1 pack cigs/day from age 18 (36 pack/yr)[+]

Alcohol/Drugs. Rare drink (wine) only, doesn't like it. No drugs

Diet. Breakfast — orange juice, 2 sweet rolls, black coffee

> Mid-morning — doughnut, coffee

> Lunch--hamburger and bun or fish sandwich, coffee

> Dinner — meat or fish, vegetable, potato, sometimes fruit, sometimes cookies

> Snacks in evening (e.g. chips, cola)

> Has almost no milk or cheese

Tests. Last Pap smear 1991, "normal." No mammograms

Immunizations. Oral polio vaccine, yr uncertain; tetanus shots × 2 in 1991, followed by a booster 1 yr later; flu vaccine 11/93, no reaction

Sleep. Generally good, average 7 hr, sometimes has trouble falling asleep, is wakened by alarm

Exercise/Leisure. "No time"

* *Hazards.* Medicines kept in unlocked medicine cabinet. Cleaning solutions, furniture polish, and Drano in unlocked cabinet below sink, Mr. N's shotgun and box of shells is in upstairs closet.

Safety. Seat belt regularly

[+] (Age 54 yr - 18 yr) × (1 pack) = 36 pk/yr.

Family History

The family history can be recorded in *outline form*, as here. The *diagram form*, not shown here, can be helpful in tracing genetic disorders.

Father died, 43, train accident

Mother died, 67, stroke, had varicose veins, headaches

One brother, 61, has high blood pressure, otherwise well

One brother, 58, apparently well but for mild arthritis

One sister, died in infancy, ?cause

Husband died, 54, heart attack

One daughter, age 33, "migraine headaches," otherwise well

One son, 31, headaches

One son, 27, well

No family history of diabetes, tuberculosis, heart or kidney disease, cancer, anemia, epilepsy, or mental illness

*Psychosocial. Born and raised in Salt Lake City, finished high school, married at age 19. Worked as clerk in store for 2 yr, then moved with husband to Capital City, had 3 children. Mr. N had a fairly steady factory job. To help with family income, Mrs. N went back to work 15 yr ago. Children have all married. 4 yr ago Mr. N died suddenly of heart attack, leaving little savings and no insurance. Finances now tight. Has moved to small apartment to be near daughter, Dorothy. Dorothy's husband, Arthur, has a drinking problem, is verbally though

not physically abusive. Mrs. N's apartment is a haven for Dorothy and her two children, Kevin, 6 yr, and Linda, 3 yr. Mrs. N. feels responsible for helping them, is tense and nervous, but denies depression. Has a few good friends but doesn't like to bother them with her family's trouble. "I'd rather keep it to myself. I don't like gossip." No church or other organizational support.

Typically up at 7:00 a.m.,, works 9:00 to 5:30, eats dinner alone. Dorothy or the children visit most evenings and weekends. Moderate number of squabbles and considerable strain

Review of Systems

* *General.* Has <u>gained</u> about <u>10 lb</u> in the past 4 yr

Skin. No rashes or other changes

Head. See present illness. No head injury

Eyes. Reading glasses for 5 yr, last checked 1 yr ago. No symptoms

Ears. Hearing good. No tinnitus, vertigo, infections

Nose, Sinuses. Occasional mild cold. No hay fever, sinus trouble

* *Mouth and Throat.* Some <u>bleeding of gums</u> recently. Last to dentist 2 yr ago. Occasional canker sore, has had one for 4 days

Neck. No lumps, goiter, pain

Breasts. No lumps, pain, discharge. Does breast self-exams sporadically

Respiratory. No cough, wheezing, pneumonia, tuberculosis. Last chest x-ray 1982, St. Mary's Hospital, normal

Cardiac. No known heart disease or high blood pressure; last blood pressure taken in 1987. No dyspnea, orthopnea, chest pain, palpitations. No ECG

* *GI*. Appetite good; no nausea, vomiting, indigestion. Bowel movement about once daily though sometimes has *hard stools for 2–3 when especially tense*; no diarrhea or bleeding. No pain, jaundice, gallbladder or liver trouble

* *Urinary*. No frequency, dysuria, hematuria, or recent flank pain; nocturia ×1, large volume. *Occasionally loses some urine* when coughs hard

Genital. Menarche at 13, regular periods, tapered off in late 40s and stopped at 49; no bleeding since; mild hot flashes and sweats then, none now

Gravida 3, para 3, living children 3. Prolonged labor during first pregnancy, otherwise normal. Little sexual interest now, not sexually active

* *Musculoskeletal*. Mild <u>aching low back pain</u> often after a long day's work; no radiation down legs; used to do back exercises, but not now. No other joint pain

* *Peripheral Vascular*. <u>Varicose veins</u> appeared in both legs during first pregnancy. Has had swollen ankles after prolonged standing for 10 yr; wears light elastic pantyhose; tried "water pill" 5 mo ago but it didn't help much; no history of phlebitis or leg pain

Neurologic. No faints, seizures, motor or sensory loss. Memory good

Hematologic. Except for bleeding gums, no easy bleeding. No anemia

Endocrine. No known thyroid trouble, temperature intolerance. Sweating average. No symptoms or history of diabetes

Psychiatric. See present illness and psychosocial

Physical Examination

Mrs. N is a short, moderately obese, middle-aged woman, walks and moves easily, responds quickly to questions. Wears no makeup but hair is fixed neatly and clothes are immaculate. Although ankles are swollen, her color is good and she lies flat without discomfort. Talks freely but is somewhat tense, with moist cold hands.

P 94, regular R 18 Temp 37.1°C(oral)

BP 164/98 right arm, lying

160/96 left arm, lying

152/88 right arm, lying (wide cuff)

Ht (without shoes) 157 cm (5'2")

Wt (dressed) 65 kg (143 lb)

Skin. Palms cold and moist, but color good. Scattered cherry angiomas over upper trunk

Head. Hair of average texture. Scalp and skull normal

Eyes. Vision 20/30 each eye. Visual fields full by confrontation. Conjunctiva pink. Sclera clear. Pupils round, regular, equal, react to light. Extraocular movements intact. Disc margins sharp. No arterial narrowing, A–V nicking

Ears. Wax partially obscures right drum. Left canal clear and drum negative. Acuity good (to whispered voice). Weber midline. ACBC

Nose. Mucosa pink, septum midline. No sinus tenderness

* *Mouth.* Mucosa pink. Several interdental papillae red and slightly swollen. Teeth in good repair. Tongue midline, with a (3 × 4 mm) shallow, white ulcer on red base, located on the undersurface near the tip; it is slightly tender but not indurated. Tonsils absent. Pharynx negative

Neck. Trachea midline. Thyroid isthmus barely palpable, lobes not felt

Lymph Nodes. Small (less than 1 cm), soft, nontender, and mobile tonsillar and posterior cervical nodes bilaterally. No auxiliary or epitrochlear nodes. Several small inguinal nodes bilaterally — soft and nontender

Thorax and Lungs. Thorax symmetrical. Good expansion. Lungs resonant. Breath sounds normal with no added sounds

* *Cardiovascular.* Jugular venous pressure 1 cm above sternal angle, with head of bed raised to 30°. Cartoid pulses normal and symmetrical. Apical impulse barely palpable in 5th left interspace 8 cm from midsternal line. Physiologic split of S_2. No S_3 or S_4. A 2/6 medium-pitched midsystolic murmur at 2nd right interspace; does not radiate to the neck. Diastole clear

Breasts. Large, pendulous, symmetrical. No masses. Nipples erect and without discharge

Abdomen. Obese, but symmetrical. Well healed right lower quadrant scar. Bowel sounds normal. Sigmoid colon slightly tender, no other masses or tenderness. Liver span 7 cm in right midclavicular line. Splenic percussion sign negative. Liver, spleen, and kidneys not felt. No CVA tenderness

* *Genitalia.* Vulva Normal. Mild *cystocele* on straining. Vaginal mucosa pink. Cervix parous, pink, without discharge. Uterus anterior, midline, smooth, not enlarged. Adenexa difficult to feel because of obesity and poor relaxation. No cervical or adnexal tenderness. Pap smears taken. Rectovaginal exam unremarkable

Rectal. No masses. Brown stool, negative for occult blood

* *Peripheral Vascular*

Pulses: 2+ <u>edema</u> of feet and ankles with 1+ edema extending up to just below knees. Moderate <u>varicosities</u> of saphenous veins bilaterally from midthigh to ankles, with spider veins on both lower legs. No stasis pigmentation or ulcers. No calf tenderness

	Radial	Femoral	Popliteal	Dorsalis Pedis	Posterior Tibial
RT	N	N	N	↓	N
LT	N	N	N	0	N

Musculoskeletal. No joint deformities. Good range of motion, in hands, wrists, elbows, shoulders, spine, hips, knees, ankles

Neurologic

Mental Status. Tense but alert and cooperative. Thought coherent. Oriented. Cognitive testing not done in detail

Cranial Nerves. See head and neck. Also —

    I — Not tested

V — Sensation intact, strength good

VII — Facial movement good

XI — Sternomastoids and trapezii strong

Motor. Normal muscle bulk and tone. Strength 5/5 throughout. Rapid alternating movements and point-to-point movements intact. Gait normal. No prontor drift

Sensory. Romberg negative. Pinprick, light touch, position, vibration, and stereognosis intact

Reflexes. (Two methods of recording may be used, depending upon personal preference; a tabular form, as shown below, or a stick figure diagram.)

	Biceps	Triceps	SUP	ABD	Knee	Ankle	PL
RT	2+	2+	2+	2+/2+	2+	1+	↓
LT	2+	2+	2+	2+/2+	2+	1+	↓

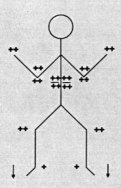

Mr. N.'s Problem List and Plan

One way to organize Mrs. N.'s problem list is shown below.

Date Problem Entered	No.	Active Problems	Inactive Problems
11/13/94	1	Migrane headaches	
11/13/94	2		Acute kidney infection
11/13/94	3	Allergy to ampicillin	
11/13/94	4	Tensions secondary to family situation, finances, and stress at work.	
11/13/94	5	Gingivitis	
11/13/94	6	Low back pain	
11/13/94	7	Varicose veins with venous insufficiency	
11/13/94	8	Cystocele with occasional stress incontinence	
11/13/94	9	Possible high blood pressure	
11/13/94	10	Diet high in calories, fat, and carbohydrates, low in calcium	
11/13/94	11	Home hazards: kitchen supplies, medicines, gun	

The list includes problems that need some attention now (such as the headaches) or may need further observation or possible future attention (such as the blood pressure and cystocele). The allergy is listed as an active problem to warn against inadvertent future prescriptions of penicillin.

A few items noted in the history and physical examination, such as canker sores and hard stools, do not appear in this problem list because they are relatively common phenomena that do not seem to demand attention. Such judgments may be wrong. Problem lists that are cluttered with relatively insignificant items, however, diminish in value. Some clinicians would undoubtedly judge this list too long; others would bring greater explicitness to problems such as "tensions," "diet," and "gingivitis."

The patient's record included notes on two of Mrs. N.'s problems:

1. *Migraine headaches*

> *Assessment.* Supporting this diagnosis are "sick headaches" in earlier life, recurrent course of headaches, their duration, their relief by cold and quiet, associated nausea and vomiting (once at least), and positive family history. Further, no related neurologic symptoms or signs. Headaches may be somewhat more frequent than typical migraine headaches, pain is usually aching rather than throbbing, and there are obvious tensions at work and at home. Tension headaches should also be considered, therefore, but the headaches fit this pattern less well.

Plan

> *Diagnostic*. Observation only. Mrs. N. to look for possible precipitating factors.
>
> *Therapeutic*. Continue aspirin as needed.
>
> *Education*. Nature of migraine discussed. Patient pleased and relieved

9. **Possible high blood pressure**

> *Assessment*. Some of apparent elevation clearly related to obese arms, and may be related to anxiety of a first visit. No evidence of target organ damage

Plan

> *Diagnostic*. Repeat BP in one month. Use wide cuff. Urinalysis Therapeutic. None now. Consider diet change on next visit.
>
> *Education*. Need for BP checks explained

Although you have insufficient information about Mrs. N.'s other problems, including her own priorities, try to develop an approach to them. What further data do you need? You have the tools to expand your knowledge of her situation further. Needed now is repetitive practice, with supervision, in using those tools.

What information do you need and how do you obtain it?

These questions appear implicitly throughout this booklet and are explored in greater detail in *A Guide to Physical Examination and History Taking, 6th Edition*, by Barbara Bates. They are care questions in any clinical practice, and will persist far beyond the initial learning experience.